DIET COOKBOOK HEMOCHROMATOSIS

A COMPLETE MEAL PLAN FOR HEMOCHROMATOSIS

KAIN POORE

Table of Contents

CHAPTER ONE

Dietary recommendations for people with hemochromatosis.

All the information you'll ever need.

Hemochromatosis causes the body to absorb an excessive amount of iron from food, resulting in an iron overload. People with hemochromatosis can lessen their symptoms and lower their risk of complications by altering their diet in certain ways.

Primary hemochromatosis and secondary hemochromatosis are both forms of the disease. Hemochromatosis can be primary or secondary. Primary hemochromatosis is inherited, while secondary hemochromatosis can be caused by liver disease or anemia.

The average daily iron absorption and loss is 1 milligram (mg). Each day, people with hemochromatosis can ingest as much as 4 mg of iron.

Excessive accumulation of iron in the organs can be toxic and result in damage. Dietary changes, however, can help you keep your iron levels at a healthy level.

The foods that a person with hemochromatosis may or may not want to eat are discussed in this article.

dietary factors

Nonheme iron, which is abundant in spinach and mushrooms, is unlikely to have a significant impact on blood iron levels.

It is the goal of treatment for hemochromatosis to bring iron levels back to normal.

When it comes to iron intake, there are other things to keep in mind. The body's ability to absorb iron is influenced, for example, by certain food components.

The following are some instances of this:

Heme iron is more easily absorbed by the body than nonheme iron. Meat, poultry, fish, and seafood contain both heme and nonheme iron, whereas the iron in plant-based foods is exclusively nonheme.

Nonheme iron absorption is enhanced by vitamin C.

• Calcium: This mineral has the ability to reduce iron absorption.

•

Nonheme iron absorption is hampered by phytates, tannins, and polyphenols, all of which are found in plant foods.

Hemochromatosis can be treated with medication and therapeutic phlebotomy, which removes blood from the body, in addition to dietary changes.

What can I eat?

People with hemochromatosis don't have any official dietary guidelines, but some foods that may help include:

a variety of fresh produce

A well-balanced diet must include plenty of fresh fruits and vegetables. Vitamins and minerals are essential for a healthy body, and they can be found in a wide variety of foods.

Iron in nonheme form is abundant in a number of vegetables and fruits, such as spinach, mushrooms, and olives. Nonheme iron is more difficult to absorb, so it is unlikely to have a significant impact on blood iron levels.

Oxidative stress can be harmful to people with hemochromatosis. In order to counteract the damage caused by oxidation, it is important to eat foods rich in antioxidants.

Vitamin E and selenium are two antioxidants found in many fruits and vegetables.

Phytochemicals, or plant compounds, are also found in plants and have anti-inflammatory and anti-viral properties. These are just a few examples of phytochemicals

Lutein can be found in dark green leafy vegetables.

The tomato pigment lycopene

in blueberries and beets anthocyanins

Protein that's low in fat and calories

Many sources of lean protein contain iron, making them an important part of a well-balanced diet.

Hemochromatosis patients do not need to avoid all animal

protein, but it is better to choose lower iron-content animal proteins like fish and chicken over higher iron-content animal proteins like red meat.

Nuts, seeds, beans, and grains are all included.

Iron absorption is reduced in grains, legumes, seeds, and nuts due to the presence of phytic acid, or phytate.

Nonheme iron absorption is decreased when phytate-rich foods like beans, nuts, and whole grains are consumed.

Consequently, the body's total iron levels may be reduced.

Coffee and tea

Tannins, which are polyphenol plant compounds, are found in both tea and coffee.

Tea and coffee's tannins may inhibit iron absorption. People with hemochromatosis can control their iron levels by drinking these beverages.

CHAPTER TWO

Foods high in calcium

Both nonheme and heme iron can be inhibited by calcium.

Calcium-rich foods include the following:

- yogurt

- milk

- cheese

- tofu

Broccoli is an example of a green leafy vegetable

Eggs

According to some studies, eggs may help prevent iron absorption.

The protein phosvitin found in eggs binds to iron and prevents it from being absorbed.

The pitfalls to watch out for

People with hemochromatosis are generally advised by doctors to avoid iron-enriched foods and supplements. The following foods should also be avoided:

The term "red meat" is used to refer to

Heme iron can be found in abundance in most red meats, including beef, lamb, and venison, to name a few. Heme levels in poultry and pork are lower than in beef.

Most red meat should be avoided by people with hemochromatosis because heme iron is so easily absorbed by the body.

Nonheme iron absorption is boosted by red meat as well.

Foods that reduce iron absorption, like red meat, may also help manage iron levels if eaten with red meat.

Shellfish that has not been cooked

Vibrio vulnificus bacteria can be found in shellfish such as mussels, oysters, and clams. Vibriosis is a serious infection caused by these bacteria.

Hemochromatosis patients are at greater risk of contracting vibriosis. As a result, it is critical that all shellfish be thoroughly cooked in order to eradicate harmful bacteria. In addition, discarding raw shellfish with open shells and avoiding eating shellfish with unopened shells after cooking can help people reduce their risk of infection.

Vitamin C is a nutrient that aids

Nonheme iron is better absorbed when vitamin C is present. As a result, vitamin C supplements should be avoided by people with hemochromatosis.

In general, the amount of vitamin C found in fruits and vegetables does not have a significant impact on iron absorption. In addition to the nutrients listed above, many of these foods are high in fiber and low in fat.

However, consuming vitamin C-rich foods and beverages along with iron-rich foods may improve absorption of iron. Hemochromatosis patients may want to avoid eating foods high in iron and low in vitamin C.

People who want to know how much daily vitamin C they need can do so by consulting their physician.

Foods enriched with nutrients

Vitamins and minerals are added to foods that have been fortified or enriched. Calcium, vitamin D, and iron are commonly added to cereals.

Those who have hemochromatosis should steer clear of iron-enriched food.

Alcohol

As a result of ingesting alcohol, the body creates compounds that harm the liver.

An increase in oxidative stress can occur when iron and alcohol are consumed in the presence of each other. Hemochromatosis may be worsened by this oxidative stress. Alcohol also boosts iron levels in the body.

People with hemochromatosis may be advised by their doctor to limit their alcohol consumption.

Is there much of an impact on this condition from a diet?

Iron absorption can be affected by diet, but the impact on hemochromatosis is unclear. Hemochromatosis patients may not need to make any dietary adjustments.

When compared to standard hemochromatosis treatments, dietary changes have only a small impact on iron levels, according to the American Association for the Study of Liver Diseases and the National Institute of Diabetes and Digestive and Kidney Diseases In small doses, diet changes can help lower iron levels. However, medication or phlebotomy are much more effective.

Hemophiliacs still need to stay away from certain foods, according to the Centers for Disease Control and Prevention and the National Heart, Lung, and Blood Institute:

- dietary supplements with vitamin C

- shellfish that has not been cooked

- excessive drinking

Treatment alternatives are available.

In most cases, hemochromatosis treatment includes the following:

Phlebotomy

At a time, one pint of blood is drawn to remove excess iron. In order to monitor iron levels, they will order regular blood tests.

Treatment with chelation

Chelation therapy uses pills or injections to remove iron from the body. Patients with conditions like anemia or heart disease may not be able to undergo blood removal, so these treatments are necessary.

Removal of iron through phlebotomy is more effective than through chelation therapies.

Hemochromatosis patients should include these foods in their diets:

1. Vegetables and fruit

Antioxidants, found in green leafy vegetables and brightly colored fruits, help prevent the production of free radicals. Iron absorption can be impaired by oxalates found in spinach. This is despite its high iron content.

Kale, rhubarb, and strawberries are also good sources of oxalates.

Inhibiting heme iron absorption has been shown to be an effect of polyphenols in fruits and vegetables like berries, plums, apples, artichokes, chicory and red onions Iron from non-heme sources like fruits and vegetables cannot be absorbed effectively.

2. Low-fat, high-protein foods.

Chicken, turkey, cod, mackerel, and salmon are all good sources of heme protein, but they are all lower in iron than red meat.

3. Grains, legumes, seeds, and nuts

Phytates, or phytic acid, found in whole grains, legumes, seeds, beans, and some nuts, can reduce the absorption of iron. They also contain a lot of fiber, which reduces the amount of non-heme iron that can be absorbed.

Eggs

In eggs, the phosphoprotein Phosvitin binds to iron and helps limit the amount of iron that the body takes in.

a cup of tea

Tannins, a common component of tea, are consumed by tea drinkers. Tea consumption, according to a 2017 review published in the journal Current Developments in Nutrition, may reduce iron absorption.

CHAPTER THREE

Dairy products

The iron content of dairy products such as milk, cheese, and yogurt is low. Additionally, they have the potential to reduce the absorption of iron from supplements and foods when taken together.

Hemochromatosis diet foods to avoid: six things to stay away from

Heme iron is more easily absorbed by the body, so avoiding foods high in heme iron is a requirement of a low-iron diet for hemochromatosis. Foods and beverages high in iron can exacerbate the symptoms of hemochromatosis.

Hemochromatosis sufferers should avoid or limit the following foods and beverages:

Foods high in vitamin C

Hemochromatosis and iron overload can both be exacerbated by consuming foods and beverages high in vitamin C, according to Dr. Singh.

Overconsumption of red meat

Heme iron, which is more readily absorbed by the body, is found in animal protein sources like beef, according to nutritionist Best. There may be no harm in including small amounts of red meat in the hemochromatosis diet if discussed with a healthcare provider or registered dietitian.

3. Seafood that has been defrosted and served raw.

Vibrio vulnificus, a bacterium found in warm saltwater, can be found in raw fish and shellfish, especially oysters. Vibriosis is a disease that can be caused by this bacterium. Vibriosis can infect anyone, but the CDC warns that people with iron overload disease, particularly those with liver involvement, are more likely to contract the infection or develop complications from it than the general population. Fever, chills, diarrhea, nausea, and vomiting are all signs to watch out for, as is an infection on the skin that is red and warm to the touch.

Beverages that contain alcohol

advises people with hemochromatosis to avoid or limit their consumption of alcohol, as it may cause liver damage. Hemorrhagic cirrhosis patients are advised to abstain from alcoholic beverages altogether until their condition improves.

Sugar

According to a 2013 study published in PLOS ONE, foods and beverages high in certain sugars can increase the absorption of non-heme iron by approximately 300 percent. There is a strong correlation between consumption of high-fructose corn syrup (HFCS) and an increased risk of cardiovascular disease. Dietary iron absorption was not enhanced by sucrose or glucose.

Foods high in iron

Iron is added to a variety of foods, including breakfast cereals. Iron overload can be triggered by consuming iron-rich fortified foods.

Fasting is good for hemochromatosis, or is it bad?

Fasting at certain times of the day or on certain days of the week is a popular eating method. Eating and fasting must be alternated in order to achieve this effect.

Intermittent fasting can be done in a variety of ways, and each method has its own set of health benefits. When it comes to fasting and hemochromatosis, there is very little research on the benefits and risks.

Summary

An iron overload is caused by the disease hemochromatosis.

To treat hemochromatosis, phlebotomy or chelation therapy can be used to remove excess iron from the blood. Vitamin C supplements, raw seafood, and excessive alcohol consumption should all be avoided.

Choosing foods that are low in iron or reduce iron absorption can also help maintain normal iron levels. Other hemochromatosis treatments, on the other hand, have been found to be more effective.

THE END